Opening the Doors to Canadian Medical Schools

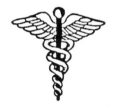

D. Roderick Elford, M.D.

Detselig Enterprises Ltd.
Calgary, Alberta

Opening the Doors to Canadian Medical Schools

© 1994 Rod Elford

Canadian Cataloguing in Publication Data

Elford, Rod, 19**

Opening the doors to Canadian medical schools

Includes bibliographical references.
ISBN 1-55059-084-7

1. Medical colleges–Canada–Entrance requirements. 2.
Medical colleges–Canada–Entrance examinations. 3. Medi-
cal colleges–Canada–Directories. I. Title.
R749.A6E43 1994   610'.71'171   C94-910317-9

Publisher's Data

*Detselig Enterprises Ltd. appreciates the financial support
for our 1994 publishing program, provided by the Department of Communications, Canada Council and the Alberta
Foundation for the Arts, a beneficiary of the Lottery Fund of
the Government of Alberta.*

Detselig Enterprises Ltd.
210, 1220 Kensington Road NW
Calgary, Alberta T2N 3P5

Edited by Sherry Wilson McEwen

Cover design by Dean MacDonald

Printed in Canada   ISBN 1-55059-084-7   SAN 115-0324

I dedicate this book to my grandfather,

John Glenn Elford

whose support was instrumental in giving me
the perseverance to see this project through to
completion.

> *If I have been able to see farther than others, it was*
> *because I stood on the shoulders of giants.*
> *– Sir Isaac Newton*

Contents

Other books in the *Life Line* series:

Prologue

The purpose of this book is to help improve your chances of getting into a Canadian medical school. During the last few years, there have been five times as many applicants to medical school as there are positions. *Opening the Doors to Canadian Medical Schools* contains up-to-date information on how the medical school selection process works, the characteristics admission committees are looking for in applicants and recommendations on how to make yourself as appealing an applicant as possible.

> To win at the admissions game,
> you must know the rules.

The ideas, words of wisdom and advice contained in this book have come from a variety of people: medical school admissions committee members, physicians and medical students. They attend and work at different medical schools, clinics and hospitals across the country. This book is an assimilation of their cumulative input and my research and personal experience with the process.

The training of the medical school gives a man his direction, points him the way, and furnishes him with a chart, fairly incomplete, for the voyage; but nothing more.
– Sir William Osler

Introduction

My name is Rod Elford and I grew up in Calgary. I enjoy participating in sports, and as a result completed an undergraduate degree in physical education (honors). I studied medicine and graduated from the University of Alberta. At present I work as a Family Medicine Resident for the District Hospital Group in Calgary.

When I applied to medical school, I found it surprising that there were no books written on how to get into a Canadian medical institution. After going through the admissions process myself, teaching MCAT orientation seminars, interviewing medical school applicants and fielding questions from many pre-med students, I decided to do some additional research. The result is this book.

If *Opening the Doors to Canadian Medical Schools* assists you in your goal to become a physician, or if you have anything to add that you feel would be helpful to other applicants, please feel free to write me at the following address:

Rod Elford
c/o 1129 - 9 St. NW
Calgary, Alberta, Canada
T2M 3K9

> *I shall pass through this world but once; any good that I can show, let me not defer it or neglect it, for I shall not pass this way again.*
> *– John Wesley*

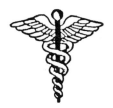

Chapter 1

Medicine as a Profession

So You Want to Be a Doctor?

You want to be a doctor? Think about it first!

Ask yourself why. Not only is this a good exercise in self-examination, but you will most likely have to answer the question during one of your medical school interviews.

Write down three reasons why you want to become a doctor. After reading this book, check and see if your answers are still the same.

Three reasons I want to become a doctor:

1. _____

   _____

2. _____

   _____

3. _____

   _____

> *Whatever you are by nature, keep to it; never desert your own line of talent. Be what nature intended you for, and you will succeed; be anything else and you will be ten thousand times worse than nothing.*
> *– Sydney Smith*

Medicine—A Good Profession?

If you have decided to become a doctor—that's great!
Medicine as a profession can provide you with one of the
most emotionally satisfying and financially rewarding
jobs you could choose. Many people would use adjectives
like "challenging," "rewarding" and "altruistic" to describe it, and there certainly are many positive qualities
attached. On the other hand, there are some "less than
positive" aspects to medicine that anyone applying for a
career in the field must consider. These include:

1. **Long training period**. The "average" licensed physician (as of 1994) will have completed three years
   of undergraduate university, four years of medical
   school and at least two years in a residency program (a resident is a doctor training in a specialty
   area). The length of residency training varies depending upon the specialty chosen, and ranges
   from two years for a family physician, to seven
   years for a cardiovascular surgeon. The total number of years of post-graduate (after high school) education needed to become a doctor: at least nine
   years, with most having completed much more.

   Personally, I did four years of undergrad, four years of
   medical school, and two years residency training in family medicine. Total time: 10 years.

2. **Expense**. To become a doctor not only takes a lot of
   time, but a lot of money. The average medical
   school graduate, who has completed three years of
   undergraduate training and four years of medical
   school, would have needed anywhere from
   $28 000 – $70 000 to finance his/her education.
   The difference in cost depends upon whether you
   lived at home with your parents, or on your own.
   (The lower value is arrived at by multiplying the

14

estimated cost of going to school while living with your parents, $4 000/year x 7 years = $28 000. The higher value is arrived at by multiplying the estimated cost of living on your own, $10 000/year x 7 years = $70 000.) The expense of becoming a doctor is formidable. Only you can decide if it is worth it.

The most common sources of income for medical students include: student loans, work, savings, money from parents, scholarships and/or bursaries. Most universities have a large number of scholarships and bursaries for students who achieve academic excellence or can demonstrate financial need. I strongly recommend investing the time to find out if you are eligible.

After graduating from medical school, you become a resident and do receive a salary. However, taking into account expenses (exams, malpractice insurance, student loans, etc.) you will not have much left over.

I lived with my parents for three of my four years of undergrad, living on my own for one year of undergrad and all four years of med school. Although I took out no loans in undergrad because I had a scholarship, I needed financial assistance in medical school. When I graduated I had $34 000 in loans. That was more than I grossed in my first year as a resident ($32 000). Although you may eventually make a lot of money as a physician ($100 000+), it takes a long time to get there. Conclusion: Expect to be poor for at least 10 years after your high-school graduation!

If you think education is expensive, try ignorance!
– Derek Bok

3. **Long hours of work**. As a student intern (a medi-
    cal student who is doing his/her in-hospital train-
    ing) or resident, it is not unusual to work 60–90
    hours a week. Most physicians work approxi-
    mately 60 hours per week. In comparison, the av-
    erage 8–5 job has a 40-hour work week. A 40-hour
    work week translates into working 8 hours a day,
    Monday to Friday. Comparatively, a physician
    would work 12 hours a day for the same five days.
    This means less free time for the physician to pur-
    sue other interests or to spend with family and
    friends.

4. **Call**. Most residents are on-call 1 in 3 or 1 in 4. This
    means every third or fourth day (including
    through the night) they are responsible for pa-
    tients. Call is usually taken from the hospital,
    meaning you sleep at the hospital the night you
    are on-call. In some rotations (surgery) it may be
    so busy that you do not sleep at all, but you are
    still expected to work the next day. Call *can* also
    be taken from home in some rotations (such as
    family medicine and psychiatry). These areas are
    usually not as busy.

    In my opinion, call is the most demanding aspect of
    medicine—not only is it tiring, but it interferes
    with your lifestyle. If you are married it means
    that every third or fourth night you may not see
    your spouse. It also makes it difficult to plan activ-
    ities in advance, or commit to an on-going activity
    on a specific day of the week.

    Generally, call is less frequent after you have com-
    pleted your residency; however, this varies consid-
    erably. The amount of call you are required to do
    depends on where you work and the number of
    other physicians in your group with whom you
    have made a deal to share call. For example, the
    only general practitioner in a small town would be

on-call every day, and could be called at any time to see patients. In contrast, a doctor who works in a large city practice with a number of other physicians may be on call once a week. How busy you are on call is often related to your specialty. Surgeons and obstetricians usually have the busiest call and may be up all night. In other specialties, like pathology and radiology, call is normally less demanding. Some nights these specialists may not even be called into the hospital.

General Trends in Medicine

In addition to the factors mentioned earlier, there are a number of general trends occurring within our society which are affecting how medicine is practised. As a result of these trends, some doctors feel the "Golden Age" of medicine has passed, and that physicians are quickly becoming "glorified civil servants." Their reasons for this opinion are:

1. **Increasing government control.** Since the vast majority of Canadian doctors' incomes are paid by the government, the government has a certain amount of control over how these funds are allocated. Within the last few years, due to the poor economic climate, large deficits, and budget cuts, all provincial governments are looking at ways to reduce health care costs. The approaches are varied and include: limiting the total amount an individual physician can bill; decreasing the compensation a new doctor can bill for a service if he/she elects to set up a clinic in an over-serviced area; decreasing all government health-service employee salaries a certain percentage; limiting the number of new doctors who can set up a practice in a province. Most provincial governments have recently enacted legislation that restricts new billing num-

bers (a number that allows a doctor to bill the government for his/her services) to physicians who have graduated from their provincial medical school or residency program. This law effectively shuts out all graduates who trained outside the province. For example, had I graduated two years ago, I could have gotten a billing number in any province in Canada. Due to restrictions (as of mid-1994) I will be able to get a billing number only in Alberta and Saskatchewan. My freedom of choice as to where I can practise medicine has been severly limited. Government control over the health care system, including physicians, is expected to increase in the future as governments attempt to further reduce health care costs and balance their budgets.

2. **Increased hospital control**. Doctors who rely on hospital personnel and equipment in order to do their jobs are finding that hospital administrators are increasingly dictating "what, where and when" they can practise. Firstly, many surgeons (who need an operating room, operating equipment and staff to assist them in surgery) do not operate as much as they would like simply because the hospital cannot afford to keep the operating rooms (OR) open. One hospital I worked in as a student intern closed down the operating rooms for an entire month, in effect putting surgeons out of work for four weeks. The doctors were simply told that the hospital did not have the money to keep the ORs open. Secondly, health service unions (nurses, cleaning staff), who outnumber doctors on staff, often have more input into how the hospital runs than physicians do, which affects what time the OR opens and when it shuts down.

3. **Decreased respect**. Many physicians feel that doctors are not as respected as they once were in the

past. Reasons for this change in public attitude are unclear but are probably due to:

- an increasing public knowledge of medical information
- a system of socialized medicine in which health care is seen as a right, not a privilege
- a decrease in community-based medical practices, and
- provincial medical associations which do not emphasize or have poor public relations.

4. **Decreased income**. Many provinces have either capped individual doctor's incomes, limited the total amount all physicians in the province can bill collectively, or simply reduced the amount a doctor can bill for a particular procedure or service. Capping means physicians are only allowed to make so much money, after which they either do not get paid for working or make only a percentage of what they usually would for the same service. At present, most physicians are paid on a fee-for-service basis (the more you work, the more you make). Many physicians foresee themselves becoming salaried (paid a specific amount of money per year) at a much lower rate than what they are making currently.

> *I never been in no situation where havin' money made it any worse.*
> *– Clinton Jones*

Table 1. Average Net Professional Incomes of Selected Groups of Taxable Self-Employed Professionals in Canada (1990)		
Profession	Number	Average Net Income* (C $)
Physicians	39 810	116 890
Dentists	9 070	100 900
Lawyers	22 710	93 220

Note: The average net income calculated for physicians includes both general practitioners (GPs) and specialists. Usually, specialists have higher incomes than GPs. They also have a longer training period.

Table 1 lists the average net income made by Canadian physicians, dentists and lawyers in 1988. While these figures show that those professionals do have a healthy income, these statistics need to be taken with a grain of salt. The tax rate for people who have incomes at this level is 30–50 percent, meaning the government takes one-third to one-half of the average net income for income tax. And, even though most doctors net more money than dentists and lawyers, they also work longer hours. On average, doctors work 60 hours a week, compared to dentists who average 40 hours a week. If physicians worked the same number of hours as dentists, they would only make $77 927 (based upon the same rate per hour). If your goal is to become rich by being a doctor, I suggest you choose a different profession. There are much easier ways to make money, and the vast majority do not require such a long and arduous training period.

One of the consequences of the decreasing independence and earning potential for physicians in Canada is that a number are moving to the United States. Although U.S. doctors do have more freedom and the potential to make more money, a downside to practising medicine in the States is the increased probability that you will be sued and the difficulty of collecting on your bills. I believe that this trend of physicians moving south will continue for the next few years.

Summary of Trends

The trends on the previous pages have been brought to your attention to help you to understand what practising medicine entails and where it is heading. I am not trying to dissuade you from becoming a doctor, or paint a gloomy picture about the future of medicine; however, these factors need to be taken into account when deciding if medicine is really the profession for you. Getting into medical school, staying in medical school, doing a residency and finally practicing medicine, is going to take a lot of time, money and hard work. Often the demands placed on you and the stress you face can be intimidating. There have been many times when I felt discouraged. I can confidently say, however, that medicine is a great profession, a profession of which I am honored to be a member. But a great profession exacts a great cost; only you can decide if it is worth it.

> *Two roads diverged in a wood, and I –*
> *I took the one less travelled by,*
> *And that has made all the difference.*
> *– Robert Frost*

21

If You're Not Sure, How Do You Find Out?

If you are not sure that you want to become a doctor, one of the best sources of information about the medical profession is to talk to someone already in the field. Your family doctor would probably enjoy discussing your interest in medicine as a future occupation. Since doctors are often extremely busy, it is best to arrange a time to talk to him or her outside of scheduled clinical hours. Do not go in for a physical and launch a barrage of questions about the medical field. I recommend phoning the office and if possible, talking to the doctor personally about arranging a time to discuss your interests. If he/she is unavailable, leave a message.

Another good source of information is medical students. Students can tell you first-hand about the trials of getting into and staying in medicine. They may not be able to tell you much about what practising medicine is really like, as they do not have the experience. If you do not know a medical student, phone a medical school near you and see if they can recommend someone for you to talk to.

What Type of Physician Should You Talk to?

Who you talk to depends entirely on what areas of medicine interest you. There are many different types of doctors. The Royal College of Physicians and Surgeons of Canada recognizes 58 different specialty areas. The type of work involved in each of the specialty areas is very different.

For example, a pathologist will spend the majority of his/her time analyzing different tissue specimens and coming up with histological diagnoses. A trauma surgeon, on the other hand, commonly sees patients who present with acute, life-threatening injuries (internal bleeding, subdural hematoma, flail chest) sustained in motor vehicle accidents. Table 2 on the following page lists all the recognized Canadian specialties.

Summary

Entrance to medical school is not a piece of cake. If you are not really sure you want to be a doctor, it is unlikely you will be motivated to do well enough to be accepted. On the other hand, if you are really determined to become a physician, this is the first step of many towards your goal.

Once you've decided to "go for it!" the following chapters offer a number of helpful hints to increase your chances of success.

> *If you don't know where you are going, you will probably end up somewhere else.*
> *– Lawrence J. Peter*

Table 2. Recognised Royal College Specialties

anatomical pathology	medical microbiology
anesthesia	medical oncology
cardiology (adult/pediatric)	neonatal medicine
cardiovascular and thoracic surgery	nephrology (adult/pediatric)
clinical immunology (adult/pediatric)	neurology (adult/pediatric)
clinical pharmacology	neuropathology
community medicine	neurosurgery
critical care medicine (adult/pediatric)	nuclear medicine
dermatology	obstetric/gynecology
diagnostic radiology	occupational medicine
emergency medicine	ophthalmology
endocrinology (adult/pediatric)	orthopedic surgery
family medicine*	otololaryngology
gastroenterology(adult/pediatric)	pediatrics
general pathology	physical medicine & rehabilitation
general surgery (adult/pediatric)	plastic surgery
geriatric medicine	psychiatry
gynecologic oncology	radiation oncology
hematology (adult/pediatric)	respiratory medicine (adult/pediatric)
hematological pathology	rheumatology (adult/pediatric)
infectious disease (adult/pediatric)	thoracic surgery
internal medicine	urology
maternal-fetal medicine	vascular surgery
medical biochemistry	

*Family medicine has its own separate college, the College of Family Physicians of Canada (CFPC).

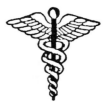

Chapter 2

Qualifying for Medical School

The "Secret" of Being Accepted into Medical School

The secret to getting into medical school is really quite simple. I learned it from a wise man who had a wealth of experience working on research and medical school selection committees.

Don't give the selection committee an excuse NOT to let you in.

It is vitally important that you understand this concept. Admissions committees do not look for candidates to admit; rather, they look for candidates who should NOT be admitted. They search for reasons to reject a candidate. The people who get into medical school are not necessarily the ones who were selected—rather they are the ones who were not rejected.

> *People at the top of the tree are those without qualifications to detain them at the bottom.*
> *– Peter Ustinov (British actor)*

Criteria Used to Select Applicants

In an American survey (no equivalent Canadian study has been done), admission officers were asked to list the sources of information they consider in processing medical school applications. Heavy importance was placed on:

- undergraduate grade-point average*
- letters of evaluation*
- medical school interview ratings*
- MCAT data*
- involvement in extracurricular activities*
- involvement in and quality of health-related experience
- breadth and difficulty of undergraduate coursework
- quality of degree-granting institution

Moderate importance was placed on:

- involvement and quality of graduate and post-graduate work
- personal comments on the application forms
- demographic factors (location of permanent address)
- involvement in undergraduate research experience

Although this was an American study, Canadian medical schools rank the importance of applicant information similarly. The criteria with asterisks (*) is definitely considered important at most Canadian educational institutions. At some Canadian schools, preferential treatment is given to applicants from the school's own province or region.

Determination of Final Ranking Order

Most Canadian medical schools divide information about their applicants into two categories, academic and non-academic. These categories are further subdivided into:

Academic	Non-academic
– undergraduate grades	– interview
	– letters of reference
– MCAT scores	– extracurricular activities
– research*	– essay

Most schools prefer the applicant to have some research experience, although it is not a major factor.

Medical schools in Canada rank the importance of the above items differently. For example, McMaster University has a tendency to place more importance on the non-academic qualities of the applicant than a school like Toronto, which is more academically orientated. Each school has its own system to arrive at a final ranking order of applicants. Some schools use a formula to convert each applicant's score into a numeric value and then rank the applicant accordingly.

Example:

Final rank order value = 0.4(GPA) + 0.2(interview) + 0.1(MCAT) + 0.1(references) + 0.1(essay) + 0.1(other) = 1/1

Each medical school will alter this formula, adding or subtracting categories, or weighting them differently. Generally, most schools give the academic category more weight. This means people with poorer marks have a higher probability of being rejected. Because competitive applicants will all have similar grades, what gives a candidate the edge in the final ranking order is how he/she performs in the *non-academic* category.

Qualifications Summary

To gain admittance to a medical school in Canada, it is to your benefit to excel in the following areas:

1. Academic requirements
2. The MCAT
3. The Essay

4. The Interview

5. Extracurricular activities

6. Reference letters

Now that you know the factors admissions committees look at in ranking applicants, the next step is to understand in depth the different parts of the application process. Read on to learn about the specifics.

> *Genius is one percent inspiration and ninety-nine percent perspiration.*
> *– Thomas Edison*

Academic Requirements

Getting good grades is a necessity if you are going to be accepted into medical school. If you are not going to commit yourself to do well academically, you are only setting yourself up for failure.

What GPA Do You Need?

Generally speaking, to get into a Canadian medical school, a student needs to have a grade point average (GPA) of 3.3 or above on the 4.0 scale. This is roughly equivalent to a B+ average (75%) or 7.5 on the 9.0 scale. The exact cut-off values vary from school to school, and year to year. For this reason, some schools do not publish minimum standards. Of the schools that do publish minimum GPAs for admittance, Calgary requires a 3.00, whereas out of province applicants to Toronto need a 3.70 (1992-93). Remember, these are the *minimum* requirements. It is possible to get into medical schools with an average lower than 3.3, but it limits the number of schools you can apply to, and greatly diminishes your chances of success. The applicants with the highest admittance rates have GPAs of 3.5 and higher.

As mentioned in the last chapter, each school calculates your GPA differently. They may use your overall average GPA (include all courses you have taken), however they are often more selective and calculate your GPA based upon: 1) your last two years, 2) your best two years, 3) marks obtained in the required pre-med courses, or any combination of these. Usually more emphasis is given to your marks in your last couple of years of university/college. (I do not know why this is the case—possibly admission committees assume that if you know you are going to apply to medicine you will make a special effort to do well.) Whatever the reason, it is a wise idea to enroll in some easier courses in your final year(s) before you apply to medical school to improve your GPA.

Why Do You Need Good Marks?

You need good marks because selection committees require some basis on which to compare candidates, and "one of the best ways to assess your intelligence is through academic grades" (quoted from a university source). Although I do not necessarily agree with the last statement, it is vital to remember that getting good grades is a *necessity*. Almost everyone you will be competing against to get into medical school will have good marks. Do not make excuses to yourself like, "I was so involved in my extra-curricular activities that my grades dropped." Other people will be involved in many activities and still get high marks.

What If You Haven't Got Good Grades?

If you have not achieved high marks, I can give you one glimmer of hope. I read about someone who got into an American medical school with a 2.0 average, but it was noted that the circumstances were exceptional. (My calculated probability of getting in with a GPA of 2.0 is about the same as winning the 6/49 lottery.) In general, though, it *is* easier to get into a medical school in the United States than in Canada.

Comparison of Acceptance Rates— Canadian Versus American

In 1992/93 there were 8 259 applicants to the 16 medical schools in Canada. The number of students admitted that year was 1 732, a success rate of 21.0%. Therefore, the odds of getting into a Canadian medical school are approximately 1 in 5. In the United States, your chances of success are greater; approximately 1 in 3 people who apply to an American medical school get accepted.

Probability of Being Accepted into Medical School

Canadian School—approx. 1 in 5 (20%)

American School—approx. 1 in 3 (33%)

Although it is easier to get into an American medical school, it is much more expensive; tuition fees vary substantially between schools, but are usually at least four times that of Canadian schools.

Some colleagues of mine who weren't accepted into a Canadian medical school went to the United States for training. Most of them completed their training south of the border, however, two transferred back to a Canadian medical school after one year. Transferring between countries is possible, but is becoming increasingly difficult. With the downsizing of Canadian medical schools, it may become impossible. If you do complete medical school in the States, it is still possible to return to Canada afterwards to do a residency, although this too is becoming more difficult.

Course Requirements

In the past, it was almost a necessity to enroll in a basic science program (chemistry, physics, biology) to get into medical school. Today, the system is much more flexible and many schools will accept students from non-science backgrounds. McMaster University will even accept students who have never taken a university science course! For the majority of schools, however, it is still necessary to take the core sciences. This includes:

- 1 full year of biology
- 1 full year of general chemistry
- 1 full year of organic chemistry
- 1 full year of physics

Most schools will *not* accept students unless they have taken these courses and many require other courses in addition, such as English, Math and Statistics. Medical schools may change their admission requirements yearly, so I advise checking the specific school's academic calendar. Interestingly, two Canadian medical schools, Calgary and McMaster, do not have any required courses; however, it is expected that the student will do some required reading during the summer prior to admittance. The minimum requirements for admittance to each Canadian medical school are listed in *Table 3. Minimum Requirements for Admittance to Canadian Medical Schools* (see p. 30). (Table 3. is taken from the *Admission Requirements to Canadian Faculties of Medicine and their Selection Policies 1993/94 & 1994/95.* The Association of Canadian Medical Colleges, Ottawa, Canada, 1992.)

Table 3. Minimum Requirements for Admittance to Canadian Medical Schools (1992–93)

University	Minimum Years of University/Grade	Required Courses
British Columbia	3 yrs./70%	Core*** & English, Math, ½ Biochemistry
Calgary*	2 yrs./ Albertans 3.0, others 3.5	Core*** & English, ½ (Zoology, Biochemistry, Psychology, Math)
Alberta**	2 yrs./ Albertans 7.0, others 8.0	Core*** & English, ½ Statistics
Saskatche-wan	2 yrs./ Sask. 70%, others 80%	Core*** & English, Humanities
Manitoba	Degree/ 3.5 for interview	Core*** & English, ½ Biochemistry
Western	3 yrs./ not available (N/A)	Core*** & 3 other non-science ½ courses
McMaster	3 yrs./B, 3.0	no required courses
Toronto	2 yrs./Ont. 3.4, others 3.7	Core*** & English
Queens	3 yrs./ N/A	Core***
Ottawa	2 yrs./3.3, B+	Core***
McGill	2 yrs./ N/A	Core*** & ½ Cell biology, Molecular biology
Montreal	2 yrs./ N/A	Standarde****
Sherbrooke	2 yrs./ N/A	Standarde****
Laval	2 yrs./ N/A	Standarde****
Dalhousie	Degree/ N/A	Bachelor's Degree
Memorial*	2 yrs./ N/A	20 courses (2 full yrs.), English

*Calgary courses are recommended, not required
**Alberta–if students apply after 2 yrs. they need min. 8.0 on 9 scale
***Core courses include 1 full yr. of: biology, physics, chemistry & organic chemistry
****Standarde courses include:BIO 310, 401; MAT 102, 103; CHM 101, 201, 202; PHY 101, 201, 301.

> *The best career advice to give to the young is, "Find out what you like doing best and get someone to pay you for doing it."*
> *— Katerine Whitehorn (journalist)*

Do You Need A Degree?

The minimum course requirements needed to enter medical school are increasing. In the past, all schools only required two years of post-graduate education for admittance. Over the last few years, there has been a trend toward selecting entrants with more educational experience. Many schools now require at least three years of university/college education and two schools, Manitoba and Dalhousie, require a university degree. As of 1995, Memorial will also expect entrants to have a degree.

The number of entrants with degrees has been steadily increasing. Table 4 (see p. 32) shows that 33.1% of the entrants to medical school in 1992/93 had degrees. This means almost one-third (573) of the 1 732 entrants to medical school in that year had degrees. This trend will continue to increase as more schools make having a degree a mandatory requirement for admittance.

> *I have never let my schooling interfere with my education.*
> *— Mark Twain*

Table 4. Total Number of 1992/93 Entrants with Degrees		
Entrants	Number of Entrants	Percentage of Total Entrants
Men with degrees	294	33.9%
Women with degrees	279	32.3%
Total entrants with degrees	573	33.1%
Total Entrants (with and without degrees): **1 732**		

What Type of Degree?

The best words of advice I can offer in regards to the degree program you choose is, *Enjoy your undergraduate program!*

University is more than a place to study—there is much more to learn than what can be found in books. Try to enjoy your university experience and develop areas of your personality outside of the academic side.

Since it is not necessary these days to take a pure science route, I recommend majoring in any field that interests you. This may mean getting a degree in Psychology, Fine Arts, or Engineering, as well as picking up the required pre-med courses. One potential disadvantage to taking a non-science route is that you may have to achieve minimally higher marks to obtain admittance to medical school than if you had stayed in sciences, say 3.60 instead of 3.50.

This is because the selection procedure is subjective. Most of the people evaluating a medical school applicant have graduated with a science degree and so tend to rank the faculty and school from which you have come according to the level of difficulty they feel should be attributed to the program. For example, they may feel that a person graduating with a degree in chemistry from McGill worked harder to obtain a 3.4 than a person who graduated in physical education from the University of Calgary. This may or may not be the case but—*that's life!* As well, taking a science major will better prepare you for writing the MCAT exam. It is really not a problem if you are not in sciences, but it does mean you will have to study harder for the MCAT.

I feel that if you enroll in courses you like, you will do better in them. Also, they will be more enjoyable. Do something you like, so that if you do not get into medical school you have another career to fall back on.

> *Just as eating contrary to the inclination is injurious to the health, so study without desire spoils the memory, and it retains nothing that it takes in.*
> *– Leonardo da Vinci*

I did an honors degree in Physical Education (specializing in biomechanics and exercise physiology). Although my pre-med major was unusual, I took all the required pre-med courses as options. Looking back, I enjoyed my undergraduate years and would not have done it any other way. If I hadn't been accepted into medical school, I likely would have become a sports therapist/trainer.

Getting Good Grades

1. Spread your classes out evenly over the year. Don't cram all your hard classes into one semester. Similarly, if you are in sciences, do not take too many courses with labs during the same term. I advise not taking more than three labs per semester.

2. Take hard classes at times when you increase the probability of doing well. This can be accomplished in a variety of ways:

a) Take a difficult class during the spring or summer, if you know that the class is easier at that time.

b) Take the class at another institution. Make sure it will be easier there and also that it is transferable.

c) Be well prepared for a difficult class.

   I took cellular biology after one semester of general biology and while taking First year chemistry. Most students had already taken one year of biology, one year of chemistry, microbiology and genetics. It's no wonder I thought the course was hard!

Course and Marks Summary

1. Strive for an average of at least 3.3 out of 4.0.

2. You must take the required courses. Generally this includes:

   • 1 year biology

   • 2 years chemistry

   • 1 year physics

   Check school calendar for specifics!

3. Take a major you enjoy–not necessarily science.

4. Evenly distribute your classes and labs.

> *To spend too much Time in Studies, is Sloth; To use them too much for Ornament, is Affection; To make Judgement wholly by their rules is the humor of a Scholar. Crafty men condemn Studies; simple men admire them; and wise men use them.*
> *– Francis Bacon*

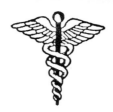

Chapter 3

The Medical College Admissions Test (MCAT)

The MCAT is a really tough exam! It takes an entire day to write and costs in the neighborhood of $150. Prepare well and do well on the exam, since you really do not want to have to write or pay for it again.

Why is It Important to Do Well?

The American Association of Medical Colleges (AAMC) booklet on the MCAT states, "The goal of the updated MCAT will be to help admissions committees predict which of their applicants will be successful in medical school." I do not necessarily agree that the MCAT can predict who will or will not be a good medical student. People who have done poorly to average on the MCAT have gone on to be stellar medical students. Still, the exam is useful as it allows medical school admissions committees to objectively evaluate candidates. This is important because it forms a common reference ground on which to compare candidates from various universities with differing standards. It is in your best interest to do well on this exam, since it is used by most schools in the selection process.

> *Examinations are formidable even to the best prepared, for the greatest fool may ask more than the wisest man can answer.*
> *– Charles Caleb Colton*

Table 5. Canadian Medical Schools Requiring the MCAT for Admission

University	MCAT Required
British Columbia	Yes
Calgary	Yes
Alberta	Yes
Saskatchewan	No
Manitoba	Yes
Western Ontario	Yes
McMaster	No
Toronto	Yes
Queens	Yes
Ottawa	Yes
McGill	Yes/No*
Sherbrooke	No
Montreal	No
Laval	No
Dalhousie	Yes
Memorial	Yes

*The five-year program at McGill does not require the MCAT to be written.

MCAT scores may not be taken into account initially, but if the admissions committee has to decide between equally qualified applicants, MCAT scores are a potential way to differentiate among candidates. Table 5 indicates which Canadian schools require the applicant to write the MCAT.

At present 11 out of the 16 Canadian medical schools require the applicant to write the MCAT. No French-speaking schools require it (as it is a English exam). Only two of the English-speaking medical schools (Saskatchewan and McMaster) do not use the exam.

The MCAT Day

The MCAT is divided into four sections; verbal reasoning, physical science, writing sample and biological sciences. Each section has a specific number of questions to be answered in an allotted period of time. Table 6 shows a summary of the MCAT day.

Table 6. Summary Table of the MCAT Day		
Section	Number of Questions	Time (mins.)
Verbal reasoning (break)	65	85 10
Physical sciences (lunch break)	77	100 60
Writing sample —essay (break)	2	60 10
Biological sciences	77	100
Total	221	7 hours

The roots of education are bitter, but the fruit is sweet.
– Aristotle

The Sections of the MCAT

1. **Verbal reasoning**. This section tests your ability to understand and evaluate information and arguments contained in prose texts. There are a number of passages, each 500–600 words long, on a variety of subjects followed by 6 to 10 multiple choice questions. All information needed to answer the questions is provided in the texts.

2. **Physical Sciences**. This section tests your reasoning in general chemistry and physics. It contains 10 or 11 problem sets, each around 250 words in length. After each set there are 4 to 8 multiple choice questions for a total of 62 questions. There are an additional 15 independent questions not related to any passage. MCAT administrators claim that the exam does not test the ability to memorize facts, and that the applicant only requires a level of knowledge of chemistry and physics equivalent to introductory university courses.

3. **Writing Sample**. The two essays you are required to write in this section are supposed to offer evidence of your writing and analytical skills. It is felt that, "adequate development of communication skills is considered a necessity for the faculty of medicine graduate, and these skills often provide the context in which the other skills of quantitative reasoning and problem solving are used." This section consists of two 30-minute essays in which the applicant is evaluated according to how well he/she does the following:

   • develops a central theme
   • presents a synthesis of concepts and ideas
   • presents ideas coherently and logically

- demonstrates clear writing, using acceptable grammar, spelling, syntax and punctuation (of a quality consistent with a timed, first-draft composition).

The topics required for essays will *not* consist of the following subject matter: biology, chemistry, physics, the medical school application process, or reasons for medicine as a career. The questions will cover topics that are within the "general experience of college students."

4. **Biological Sciences**. This section tests reasoning in biologic and organic chemistry. This section includes 10 to 11 problem sets followed by 4 to 8 multiple choice questions for a total of 62 questions. There are an additional 15 independent questions not related to any passage. Each passage is around 250 words long. Questions do not assess rote memorization of facts, rather they test concept and problem-solving ability. The level of knowledge required is comparable to introductory university level biology.

Although test administrators say you do not need to memorize facts to do the test, they do not tell you that if you have memorized a number of facts it definitely helps. It only makes sense; if you know a fact you can answer a question more quickly than if you have to take the time to figure it out. This is beneficial since you will most likely feel rushed for time during the exam.

> *We do not know one millionth of one percent about anything.*
> *– Thomas A. Edison*

What Do You Need to Score on the Exam?

The MCAT exam score is based on a 15-point scale, with the high end at 15 and the low end at 1. Each of the physical, biological and verbal reasoning sections are marked out of 15. The essays are marked a bit differently. A 6-point scale is used by two separate readers, with the scores averaged and converted to a letter grade. Everyone who writes the exam at the same time you do (approximately 25 000 people) is rank-ordered according to their scores. That means that the top people (those in the 99 percentile) get 15. Then, depending on their percentile rank, the rest of the people are assigned a corresponding number.

Ideally, you want to get an average score of 9 out of 15, or higher. Below are the MCAT scores of three hypothetical students who took the exam, and an evaluation of their performance. Scores are given in the following order: physical science, biological science, verbal reasoning.

MCAT Scores for Three Hypothetical Applicants

Applicant	Marks	Average
JOE	8,4,6	6
BOB	13,8,6	9
MARY	10,9,8	9

Joe has done poorly, getting an average of 6 on the exam. His performance would be considered unsatisfactory by admissions committees and this would decrease his chances of getting into medical school. Bob and Mary have both achieved an average of 9 on the exam, which is an acceptable score. Although their average scores are identical, Mary was more consistent in her performance. Bob, who did very well in physical sciences with 13, only received a 6 in verbal reasoning. Generally, committees prefer to see an even distribution of marks (Mary's 10,9,8) rather than more widely-distributed numbers (Bob's 13,8,6).

Average MCAT Scores

Table 7 shows that the average exam score for all applicants who wrote the MCAT was 8.55. Those candidates who received one offer of admission to a Canadian medical school on average did significantly better, scoring 9.44. Those candidates who did not receive any offers of admission scored significantly below average, with 8.11. Obviously, people who get into medical school do better than average on the MCAT. You want to be one of those people!

Table 7. 1992/93 Average MCAT Scores of Successful and Unsuccessful Applicants			
Subject	Average Scores of all applicants	One offer of Admission	No offers of Admission
Biological Science	8.77	9.75	8.27
Physical Science	8.66	9.54	8.21
Verbal Reasoning	8.23	9.03	7.86
Exam average (3 subjects)	8.55	9.44	8.11

Canadian Medical Education Statistics 1993. Vol. 15. The Assoc. of Canadian Medical Colleges, Ottawa, Canada, 1993. p. 154,155

Note: These values are only averages, meaning some people who got into medical school had an exam average above 9.44, while others had lower scores.

How to Prepare for the MCAT

1. Take University-level Courses

One of the best ways to prepare for the MCAT is to take university courses that cover the basic biological, chemical and physical sciences, and an English course. If possible take these courses the year you write the exam. Since you will already be studying for those courses it decreases the amount of extra time you have to study for the MCAT. Make note that the semester you write the MCAT you will probably spend more time studying than you ever have. Plan to be in the library a lot.

2. MCAT Student Manual and Other Manuals

The MCAT Student Manual gives descriptions of the content and cognitive skills assessed on the exam. It also has examples of full length practice tests. I found the MCAT Student Manual extremely helpful. Half of doing well on any exam is knowing what to expect. The manual familiarizes you with the exam format and style of questions used in the MCAT examination. The MCAT Student Manual should be available at your university bookstore. You can also purchase the booklet directly by phoning (202) 828-0523, or write to:

Membership and Subscriptions
Association of American Medical Colleges
One Dupont Circle, N.W.
Washington, D.C. 20036

In addition to the MCAT Student Manual, there are a number of other good manuals put out by private publishers. These manuals should also be available at your university or college bookstore. I cannot recommend one specific manual for you to purchase, since what is available across the country in bookstores will vary. I suggest asking a staff person at the university bookstore which manual has been the most popular, or talking to medical students in your area about which one they liked best. The books I have used in my MCAT seminars are:

- Barron's MCAT (how to prepare for the Medical College Admission Test). (Seibel, R. and Guyer, Kenneth E. Toronto: Barrons Educational Series)
- Arco MCAT, revised and enlarged. (Solomon, L. and Bramson, S. New York: Arco Publishing)

3. **MCAT Prep Courses**

There are a number of MCAT courses you can register in to help prepare you for the exam. All of the courses I have looked into give statistics indicating that their students do better than average on the exam. I did not take one of these courses, but friends who did believed that they felt more relaxed writing the exam than they would have if they had not taken the course. I am not sure if their decreased level of anxiety was due to taking the course or to the time they put in studying. One drawback is the expense ($500+). Most companies that offer MCAT prep courses hold classes on university campuses, starting two months before the exam. College/university counsellors should be able to give you additional information. Personally, I do not think they are worth the money.

*Important Note: Part of doing well on an exam is knowing what to expect. Whatever way you can, either by purchasing a manual or taking a course, **practice with old exams**! It is also a good idea to time yourself at least once when writing a practice exam, since you will be time limited during the actual test. Not only do you have to know your material, you must be able to answer quickly.*

The most stressful aspect of the MCAT for me was how rushed I felt. During the first section of the exam, I thought I was cruising through the questions, but I didn't finish them all before the buzzer went and I had to put my pencil down and close the test booklet.

When to Write the MCAT

The MCAT is administered twice a year, once in the spring (April) and again in the fall (September). It is recommended that you write the MCAT in the spring 1 and 1/2 years (18 months) before you plan to enter medical school. For example, you would take the MCAT in the spring of 1992 to enter medical school in the fall of 1993. If you wait until the fall, there is only a short period of time between receiving your MCAT test marks and application deadlines for medical schools (which are a year in advance). Taking the test in the spring decreases the probability that a procedural problem will prevent the completion of your application. Also, during the summer, it is unlikely that you will cover material relevant to the exam, in which case you would be poorly prepared for the exam in the fall. An exception to this rule would be if you were taking spring/summer science courses. In this case, it might be better to wait until the fall. Finally, taking the test in the spring means that if you do poorly, you have the option to rewrite the exam before medical school application deadlines.

It is best to write the MCAT soon after you have completed the basic sciences, so that the material is still fresh in your mind. For most science students this is in their second year. It is a good idea to write the MCAT at this time even if you decide to complete a degree before entering medicine. Finally,

Send for your MCAT package early—December or January for the spring exam.

MCAT packages are available at most medical schools, or can be acquired directly from:

MCAT Membership and Subscriptions
Association of American Medical Colleges
One Dupont Circle, N.W.
Washington, D.C.
20036 U.S.A.

I did not follow any of these recommendations because I didn't know about them. I wrote the exam in the fall, a year and a half after taking the core science courses, having spent the summer working, and studied for only two weeks. Although I did well enough to get into medical school, I strongly suggest following the recommendations. I know it will make your life easier and severely reduce the level of stress you feel.

Helpful Hints for the MCAT:

1. If you are a slow reader, take a speed-reading course. This will be helpful not only for the exam but for any reading/studying you have to do in the future.

2. Start studying two months in advance of the test, with a recommended 1 1/2–2 hours studying per day. (If you take a MCAT prep course this is approximately the amount of time they expect you to put in.) The amount of material you have to know is too great for you to learn in one or two days. Spread it out and pace yourself.

3. Try to get a good night's rest before the exam. It is more important to get a good rest and be awake for the exam than to cram that extra few hours the night before.

Summary for MCAT

1. Get familiar with the exam style and questions i.e. buy a manual or attend a course (I suggest the manual, it's cheaper).

2. Study adequately for the exam—start two months before.

3. Aim for an average score of 9 out of 15, or higher.

4. Write the MCAT in the spring. It is best to write it at least 18 months before you plan to enter medical school.

5. Apply early to get your MCAT package (December to write the spring exam).

6. Try to get a good night's sleep before the test.

> *The art of medicine consists of amusing the patient*
> *while Nature cures the disease.*
> *– Voltaire*

Chapter 4

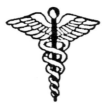

The Essay

Most medical schools require that each applicant write an essay. It is felt that an essay gives the admissions committee members insight into a candidate's character, as well as a chance to evaluate his or her writing ability. It is important that you do two things when writing the essay:

1. Answer the question.
2. Answer in the allotted space.

Although it may seem obvious to say, "Answer the question," some people don't, they just think they do. Make sure you understand what is being asked. It is a good idea to request that a friend give you some input on what he/she thinks the question is about, and some ideas on how to answer it. Even if you do stick to the topic, it is likely you will feel that the allotted space for your response is inadequate. However, staying within the allotted space is necessary as extra pages *will not be read*. Typing your response (since it is usually smaller than the written equivalent) should give you a few extra lines, plus make your essay look more professional.

> *People will sit up and take notice of you if you will sit up and take notice of what makes them sit up and take notice.*
> *— Frank Romer*

It is vitally important to realize that the people who read your essay will have read a number of essays before yours. Think for a moment how you would feel after reading hundreds of "Doctor-Wanna-Be" essays. You would probably be a little bored, not because they were bad essays, but because of the sheer volume. Make sure that your essay breaks up the monotony and is memorable. But if you are going to make it memorable, it should be remembered in a *positive way*!

Make Your Essay Memorable

My first suggestion is to start thinking about your essay a few weeks before it is due. **Do not leave it until the last minute!**

Everyone who is applying to a specific medical school will be answering the same questions. Therefore, it is possible that a large number of people will have similar answers.

For example, if one of the questions you are asked is, "Why do you want to go into medicine?" I can guarantee that most answers will include a variation of the following: a) "It's a challenge", b) "I want to make the world a better place", c) "I'm interested in learning about the human body." These are valid answers but generic. Personalize your response. **Try to incorporate personal examples into your essay, thereby making it an essay that no one else could write**. For example, tell the reader what specific experience caused you to start thinking about medicine, (e.g.) visiting a third world country or working at a nursing home. Use concrete, specific examples. Another effective technique is to demonstrate through examples in your life, qualities that are desirable in a physician, such as leadership, integrity, interpersonal skills.

Start your essay with an exciting and interesting introduction, something to catch the reader's attention and stand out from the other applicants' essays. This could be a favorite quote or some unusual aspect about yourself. Spend some time thinking about how you will capture the reader's attention. Once you have the reader's attention, state what you want the reader to know in simple and concrete terms. Make sure every word counts and that unnecessary words are omitted. **Remember to answer the question**. Finally, end with a strong conclusion. Although this may sound simple, writing a good essay is hard work. You will need many drafts before you have a quality, finished copy.

> *What is written without effort is in general read*
> *without pleasure.*
> *– Samuel Johnson*

Make Your Essay Easy to Read

Almost as important as what you say in your essay, is the way it looks on the page. As an English teacher I know says, "It should be neat and tidy and pleasing to the eye." It only makes sense—you too would appreciate the essays to be as easy to read as possible. This further emphasizes that everything you send in should be typed.

When you have completed your essay, have a friend (preferably someone who writes well) check it for spelling and grammatical errors. The essay may be the only personal item of yours that an admissions committee member sees. You do not want him/her to think that you did not care enough about your application to proof read it for errors.

Here are five guidelines on how to write (by George Orwell, author of *1984* and *Animal Farm*):

1. Never use a long word where a short one will do.
2. If it is possible to cut out a word, always cut it out.

3. Never use the passive [voice] where you can use the active.

4. Never use a foreign phrase, a scientific word or jargon words if you can think of an everyday equivalent.

5. Break any of these rules sooner than say anything barbarous.

— taken from *Politics and the English Language*

Unless one is a genius, it is best to aim at being intelligible.
— Sir Anthony Hope Hawkins (novelist)

What to Include in Your Essay

Most medical schools require the applicant to answer a specific question(s). However, if the essay question is non-specific, but is open-ended, (e.g.) "Tell us about yourself," the following would be useful to include in your response:

- reasons for wanting to become a doctor
- committees or organizations you participated in, and at what level (vice-president, secretary)
- related extra-curricular activities
- work experience
- what you have learned from your non-academic activities
- reasons for wanting to attend that particular school
- what qualities you have to offer the program

What Style to Use

Of all the essays I wrote, the ones that got the best results were written in a traditional autobiographical style: *My name is Rod Elford. I was born September 16, 1967 in Calgary, Alberta. Ever since I was a child . . .* The essays I wrote from a less traditional standpoint (one had Oprah Winfrey interviewing me on her talk show) did not fare as well. I do not know what the admissions committee thought of the latter one, but I was not asked to interview at that school. Medical people are generally conservative. It all goes back to *not* giving them a reason to reject you.

Make Your Essay Stand Out

Most applicants type their essays on standard white 8 ½" x 11" paper. One simple way to make your essay stand out is to use a heavier, watermark paper in beige, buff or some other subtle color. It is a bit more expensive than standard paper but I believe worth the money. I would advise against anything too flashy, i.e. no fluorescent pink!

If you are required to type your essay onto a standard form, there are three options you may want to try. The easiest way would be to take your essay already typed on watermark paper and glue it to the form. Better yet, you could photocopy the form onto the watermark paper and then type onto your new "form." Finally, you could type the essay onto the standard form but use a different color ink. I suggest brown. This is a subtle yet effective way to make your essay stand out.

> *It is difficult to say common things in an original way.*
> *– Horace (65-8 BC)*

On-the-Spot Essays

Most medical schools require that you write an essay to accompany your initial application. Some may not require you to write an essay until you have been selected from a larger body of applicants. Finally, a few schools do not require that you write an essay until you are at the school interviewing. These are the "on-the-spot" essays. I found writing on-the-spot essays exceedingly stressful. Two points that may help reduce your anxiety when writing these essays are:

1. You can apply most of the points mentioned in this section (intended for the essay you write at home) to the on-the-spot essay.

2. The purpose of the spontaneous essay is to test whether or not you can communicate in English, versus how well you can write. They are not looking for a literary genius; they are not looking for Shakespeare! With this in mind:

a) Try to relax.

b) Organize your thoughts and make an outline.

c) Write down your ideas in a clear and logical manner.

d) If you can think of a relevant quotation or witty remark, use it at the beginning of your essay to get the reader's attention.

> *Nothing in the affairs of men is worthy of great anxiety.*
> *– Plato*

Summary for Essay

1. Answer the question.

2. Stay within the required length.

3. Make your essay memorable by incorporating personal examples. Have an exciting, attention-getting introduction, a logical, clear middle and a strong ending.

4. Make sure it looks neat and tidy on the page (it's typewritten). Have another person check it over for errors.

> *A man may write at any time, if he will set himself doggedly to it.*
> *– Samuel Johnson*

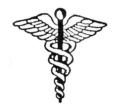

Chapter 5

The Interview

The interview may be the first and only chance the admission committee members have to meet with you. For this reason, it is important to make a good impression. In essence, you are selling a product—yourself. Like any good salesperson, you must know your product and present it in the most favorable light. You must convince your interviewers that they need you, or at least make sure they do not find any reason to reject you.

Making a good first impression is not easy; it requires effort. There are a number of ways you can prepare yourself for an interview that will increase the probability that your interview will receive a positive evaluation. A good first impression cannot be left to chance.

> *First impressions are the most lasting.*
> *– proverb*

Schools Requiring an Interview

Almost all medical schools in Canada require an interview before you are accepted. The weighting of the interview varies—for some schools it is simply a formality, at others it determines who gets accepted. If you do get an interview it means you have been selected from a larger group of applicants. It means you have passed the first hurdle.

Table 8. Canadian Medical Schools Requiring Interviews	
University	Interview Required
University of British Columbia	Yes
Calgary	Yes
Alberta	Yes
Saskatchewan	Yes
Manitoba	Yes
Western	Yes
McMaster	Yes
Toronto	not mandatory*
Queens	Yes
Ottawa	Yes
McGill	Yes
Sherbrooke	not mandatory*
Montreal	Yes
Laval	not mandatory*
Dalhousie	Yes
Memorial	not mandatory*

*These schools do not require that all entrants to their program have an interview; however, applicants that are asked to interview must attend if they wish to be admitted to the Faculty of Medicine.

How to Decrease Interview Stress

Sitting in the waiting room before a medical school interview can be one of the most stressful times in your life. You may feel as Sir Winston Churchill did when he said, "I felt as if I were walking with destiny, and that all my past life had been but a preparation for this hour and this trial."

> *Do you suppose I could buy back my introduction to you?*
> *– Groucho Marx*

The key to decreasing your stress and having a good interview is to BE PREPARED. Be prepared mentally and physically, and this will substantially increase your probability of success. Mental preparation involves anticipating potential questions, knowing your interviewer and/or school and practising your interview personality. The physical aspect involves presenting yourself in the best possible light, dressing for success and being mentally alert. Both these key areas are discussed in more depth in the following pages.

> *Successful salesmanship is 90% preparation and 10% presentation.*
> *– Bertrand R. Canfield*

Questions You May Be Asked

There are thousands of things the interviewer(s) could talk about. Try to think of what they may ask, and prepare mentally to respond to it. Below is a list of commonly-asked questions. Familiarize yourself with each question, and think about how you would answer it. Spend some time trying to predict other potential questions.

Potential Interview Questions

- Why do you want to be a doctor?
- Who influenced you in your decision?
- What type of experience do you have in the health profession?
- Why do you think you would be a good doctor?
- Why do you want to attend _____ (the school you are being interviewed at)?
- What are some ways you would improve the medical system in Canada?

Be familiar with current events! They will likely ask you about some major event that happened within the previous week just to make sure you're in touch with reality.

Be familiar with names of people who effect the medical profession, i.e. Federal and Provincial Ministers of Health.

If you did research, be ready to discuss it.

> *Picture in your mind the able, earnest, useful person*
> *you desire to be, and the thought you hold is hourly*
> *transforming you into that particular individual . . .*
> *– Elbert Hubbard*

Often they ask specifics from your resume (review it before the interview).

Think about your position on a number of ethical issues (abortion, euthanasia, patient-assisted suicide, and legalizing drugs). Ethical questions are popular and will likely be asked during your interview(s).

If you are unfamiliar with ethical issues in medicine, it would be advantageous to read a book or take a course on the subject. This will allow you to familiarize yourself with some of the current issues and form an opinion about them. Additionally, in the Appendix at the back of this book, I have included the Hippocratic Oath, the Canadian Medical Association Code of Ethics and the Medical Student Code of Ethics. Reviewing these would also be beneficial.

Know Your Interviewer(s)

If you can—either by phoning the school or talking to other students—find out who will be interviewing you (name, occupation, position), this information can be very helpful. For instance, you may find that either you or your family know your interviewer(s), or that the person works in an area that interests you. Always look for something you have in common with the interviewer, or an impressive accomplishment of the interviewer's. You may be able to bring this up in the conversation. People are always impressed if you know something about them, and love to talk about themselves. Other areas that could be useful are: research interests, sports, music, where the person was born/lived, school they attended, and so on. If you do not find out anything about your interviewer(s), or feel uncomfortable about introducing personal facts into the interview, that's fine. Knowing your interviewer is not essential, just helpful.

Know the School

If you cannot find out anything about the interviewer, it may be advantageous to know something about the school at which you will be interviewed. This information can be discovered by talking to medical students at that institution or by reading the school paper. It only makes sense to learn as much as possible about the school and its program, as this information will be invaluable if you are offered admission to more than one school. It will help you make an informed decision about whose offer of admission you will accept. Also, being able to tell the interviewers that you were impressed with the program after talking to students there shows that you have initiative and a real interest in the school.

Do the Interviewer(s) Know about You?

It is helpful to know how much your interviewer(s) know about you. At some schools, the interviewer has read your essay, resume and application form. At other schools, they know nothing about you.

In the first type of interview, they will ask you questions to find out about your personality and character traits. Additionally, they will likely refer to your resume and ask pointed questions about specific things you have done. In this case, know your resume in depth.

In the second type of interview, be prepared to tell the interviewer as much about yourself as you can in the allotted time. This means integrating important personal information into your answers. For example, if an interviewer asks you to describe one of your positive qualities you may respond, "I feel one of my character strengths is being an effective leader. During my undergraduate program, I was the President of the Green Club, a student organization dedicated to improving the quality of the environment both on and off campus." The interviewee not only answered the question, but expanded upon it. He gave a concrete example from his life of a leadership position he had held. This is a much better response than simply saying, "One of my positive qualities is that I am an effective leader."

Expanding your answer may give your interviewer fuel for the next question. In the above example, the interviewer may ask the applicant what the Green Club accomplished while he was president, or what activities the club was involved in. Hopefully, the candidate would feel comfortable answering those types of questions. When at all possible, try to direct the conversation so that the interviewer cannot help but ask you questions you are comfortable answering and which show your best side.

> *Knowledge is power – if you know it*
> *about the right people.*
> *– Chuang-Tzu*

Practise Your Interview Personality

Although it may seem awkward, I recommend practising your interview personality. In the same way you will practise old MCAT questions, go through a few mock interviews. Have someone who can be objective pretend to be the interviewer. It is best to have someone familiar with the medical school interview process, such as a doctor or counsellor. I had my father, who is a doctor and who has been on the admissions committee at the University of Calgary medical school, quiz me. Practise with interviewers of all types—mean, friendly, indifferent. Make sure the person doing the interviewing is as authentic as possible. If you are really keen, wear similar clothing to what you intend to wear during the interview. Studies have shown that people who practise in situations similar to the ones they will perform in, do better.

Psyche Yourself Up

Assure yourself that you are a wonderful person and deserve to be a medical student. Think to yourself, "If I wasn't good enough to be here, I wouldn't be." Obviously, the admissions committee feels that of all the people who applied to their school, you are worthy of being interviewed. Reaffirm to yourself before the interview that you look great. You may want to briefly check yourself out in a nearby bathroom mirror, or take a hand pocket mirror and sneak a peak before you enter. If you know you look your best, you will be more confident.

> *And, above all things, never think you're not good enough yourself. A man should never think that. My belief is that in life people will take you very much at your own reckoning.*
> *– Anthony Trollope*

Prepare Physically

Being prepared physically is just as important as being prepared mentally. Even if you have done all your homework—anticipated every question and know everything about your interviewer—you need to package yourself appropriately. Admissions committees, including those with student members, like to see a candidate who has made an effort to look good; according to societal norms this means a business-like appearance. Being prepared physically includes:

Course Requirements

In the past, it was almost a necessity to enroll in a basic science program (chemistry, physics, biology) to get into medical school. Today, the system is much more flexible and many schools will accept students from non-science backgrounds. McMaster University will even accept students who have never taken a university science course! For the majority of schools, however, it is still necessary to take the core sciences. This includes:

- 1 full year of biology
- 1 full year of general chemistry
- 1 full year of organic chemistry
- 1 full year of physics

Most schools will *not* accept students unless they have taken these courses and many require other courses in addition, such as English, Math and Statistics. Medical schools may change their admission requirements yearly, so I advise checking the specific school's academic calendar. Interestingly, two Canadian medical schools, Calgary and McMaster, do not have any required courses; however, it is expected that the student will do some required reading during the summer prior to admittance. The minimum requirements for admittance to each Canadian medical school are listed in *Table 3. Minimum Requirements for Admittance to Canadian Medical Schools* (see p. 30). (Table 3. is taken from the *Admission Requirements to Canadian Faculties of Medicine and their Selection Policies 1993/94 & 1994/95*. The Association of Canadian Medical Colleges, Ottawa, Canada, 1992.)

Table 3. Minimum Requirements for Admittance to Canadian Medical Schools (1992–93)

University	Minimum Years of University/Grade	Required Courses
British Columbia	3 yrs./70%	Core*** & English, Math, ½ Biochemistry
Calgary*	2 yrs./ Albertans 3.0, others 3.5	Core*** & English, ½ (Zoology, Biochemistry, Psychology, Math)
Alberta**	2 yrs./ Albertans 7.0, others 8.0	Core*** & English, ½ Statistics
Saskatche-wan	2 yrs./ Sask. 70%, others 80%	Core*** & English, Humanities
Manitoba	Degree/ 3.5 for interview	Core*** & English, ½ Biochemistry
Western	3 yrs./ not available (N/A)	Core*** & 3 other non-science ½ courses
McMaster	3 yrs./B, 3.0	no required courses
Toronto	2 yrs./Ont. 3.4, others 3.7	Core*** & English
Queens	3 yrs./ N/A	Core***
Ottawa	2 yrs./3.3, B+	Core***
McGill	2 yrs./ N/A	Core*** & ½ Cell biology, Molecular biology
Montreal	2 yrs./ N/A	Standarde****
Sherbrooke	2 yrs./ N/A	Standarde****
Laval	2 yrs./ N/A	Standarde****
Dalhousie	Degree/ N/A	Bachelor's Degree
Memorial*	2 yrs./ N/A	20 courses (2 full yrs.), English

*Calgary courses are recommended, not required
**Alberta–if students apply after 2 yrs. they need min. 8.0 on 9 scale
***Core courses include 1 full yr. of: biology, physics, chemistry & organic chemistry
****Standarde courses include:BIO 310, 401; MAT 102, 103; CHM 101, 201, 202; PHY 101, 201, 301.

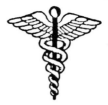

Chapter 2

Qualifying for Medical School

The "Secret" of Being Accepted into Medical School

The secret to getting into medical school is really quite simple. I learned it from a wise man who had a wealth of experience working on research and medical school selection committees.

Don't give the selection committee an excuse NOT to let you in.

It is vitally important that you understand this concept. Admissions committees do not look for candidates to admit; rather, they look for candidates who should NOT be admitted. They search for reasons to reject a candidate. The people who get into medical school are not necessarily the ones who were selected—rather they are the ones who were not rejected.

> *People at the top of the tree are those without qualifications to detain them at the bottom.*
> *– Peter Ustinov (British actor)*

Criteria Used to Select Applicants

In an American survey (no equivalent Canadian study has been done), admission officers were asked to list the sources of information they consider in processing medical school applications. Heavy importance was placed on:

- undergraduate grade-point average*
- letters of evaluation*
- medical school interview ratings*
- MCAT data*
- involvement in extracurricular activities*
- involvement in and quality of health-related experience
- breadth and difficulty of undergraduate coursework
- quality of degree-granting institution

Moderate importance was placed on:

- involvement and quality of graduate and post-graduate work
- personal comments on the application forms
- demographic factors (location of permanent address)
- involvement in undergraduate research experience

Although this was an American study, Canadian medical schools rank the importance of applicant information similarly. The criteria with asterisks (*) is definitely considered important at most Canadian educational institutions. At some Canadian schools, preferential treatment is given to applicants from the school's own province or region.

Determination of Final Ranking Order

Most Canadian medical schools divide information about their applicants into two categories, academic and non-academic. These categories are further subdivided into:

present with acute, life-threatening injuries (internal bleeding, subdural hematoma, flail chest) sustained in motor vehicle accidents. Table 2 on the following page lists all the recognized Canadian specialties.

Summary

Entrance to medical school is not a piece of cake. If you are not really sure you want to be a doctor, it is unlikely you will be motivated to do well enough to be accepted. On the other hand, if you are really determined to become a physician, this is the first step of many towards your goal.

Once you've decided to "go for it!" the following chapters offer a number of helpful hints to increase your chances of success.

> *If you don't know where you are going, you will*
> *probably end up somewhere else.*
> *– Lawrence J. Peter*

Table 2. Recognised Royal College Specialties

anatomical pathology	medical microbiology
anesthesia	medical oncology
cardiology (adult/pediatric)	neonatal medicine
cardiovascular and thoracic surgery	nephrology (adult/pediatric)
clinical immunology (adult/pediatric)	neurology (adult/pediatric)
clinical pharmacology	neuropathology
community medicine	neurosurgery
critical care medicine (adult/pediatric)	nuclear medicine
dermatology	obstetric/gynecology
diagnostic radiology	occupational medicine
emergency medicine	ophthalmology
endocrinology (adult/pediatric)	orthopedic surgery
family medicine*	otololaryngology
gastroenterology(adult/pediatric)	pediatrics
general pathology	physical medicine & rehabilitation
general surgery (adult/pediatric)	plastic surgery
geriatric medicine	psychiatry
gynecologic oncology	radiation oncology
hematology (adult/pediatric)	respiratory medicine (adult/pediatric)
hematological pathology	rheumatology (adult/pediatric)
infectious disease (adult/pediatric)	thoracic surgery
internal medicine	urology
maternal-fetal medicine	vascular surgery
medical biochemistry	

*Family medicine has its own separate college, the College of Family Physicians of Canada (CFPC).

on-call every day, and could be called at any time to see patients. In contrast, a doctor who works in a large city practice with a number of other physicians may be on call once a week. How busy you are on call is often related to your specialty. Surgeons and obstetricians usually have the busiest call and may be up all night. In other specialties, like pathology and radiology, call is normally less demanding. Some nights these specialists may not even be called into the hospital.

General Trends in Medicine

In addition to the factors mentioned earlier, there are a number of general trends occurring within our society which are affecting how medicine is practised. As a result of these trends, some doctors feel the "Golden Age" of medicine has passed, and that physicians are quickly becoming "glorified civil servants." Their reasons for this opinion are:

1. **Increasing government control**. Since the vast majority of Canadian doctors' incomes are paid by the government, the government has a certain amount of control over how these funds are allocated. Within the last few years, due to the poor economic climate, large deficits, and budget cuts, all provincial governments are looking at ways to reduce health care costs. The approaches are varied and include: limiting the total amount an individual physician can bill; decreasing the compensation a new doctor can bill for a service if he/she elects to set up a clinic in an over-serviced area; decreasing all government health-service employee salaries a certain percentage; limiting the number of new doctors who can set up a practice in a province. Most provincial governments have recently enacted legislation that restricts new billing num-

bers (a number that allows a doctor to bill the government for his/her services) to physicians who have graduated from their provincial medical school or residency program. This law effectively shuts out all graduates who trained outside the province. For example, had I graduated two years ago, I could have gotten a billing number in any province in Canada. Due to restrictions (as of mid-1994) I will be able to get a billing number only in Alberta and Saskatchewan. My freedom of choice as to where I can practise medicine has been severly limited. Government control over the health care system, including physicians, is expected to increase in the future as governments attempt to further reduce health care costs and balance their budgets.

2. **Increased hospital control**. Doctors who rely on hospital personnel and equipment in order to do their jobs are finding that hospital administrators are increasingly dictating "what, where and when" they can practise. Firstly, many surgeons (who need an operating room, operating equipment and staff to assist them in surgery) do not operate as much as they would like simply because the hospital cannot afford to keep the operating rooms (OR) open. One hospital I worked in as a student intern closed down the operating rooms for an entire month, in effect putting surgeons out of work for four weeks. The doctors were simply told that the hospital did not have the money to keep the ORs open. Secondly, health service unions (nurses, cleaning staff), who outnumber doctors on staff, often have more input into how the hospital runs than physicians do, which affects what time the OR opens and when it shuts down.

3. **Decreased respect**. Many physicians feel that doctors are not as respected as they once were in the

18

estimated cost of going to school while living with your parents, $4 000/year x 7 years = $28 000. The higher value is arrived at by multiplying the estimated cost of living on your own, $10 000/year x 7 years = $70 000.) The expense of becoming a doctor is formidable. Only you can decide if it is worth it.

The most common sources of income for medical students include: student loans, work, savings, money from parents, scholarships and/or bursaries. Most universities have a large number of scholarships and bursaries for students who achieve academic excellence or can demonstrate financial need. I strongly recommend investing the time to find out if you are eligible.

After graduating from medical school, you become a resident and do receive a salary. However, taking into account expenses (exams, malpractice insurance, student loans, etc.) you will not have much left over.

I lived with my parents for three of my four years of undergrad, living on my own for one year of undergrad and all four years of med school. Although I took out no loans in undergrad because I had a scholarship, I needed financial assistance in medical school. When I graduated I had $34 000 in loans. That was more than I grossed in my first year as a resident ($32 000). Although you may eventually make a lot of money as a physician ($100 000+), it takes a long time to get there. Conclusion: Expect to be poor for at least 10 years after your high-school graduation!

> *If you think education is expensive, try ignorance!*
> *– Derek Bok*

3. **Long hours of work**. As a student intern (a medical student who is doing his/her in-hospital training) or resident, it is not unusual to work 60–90 hours a week. Most physicians work approximately 60 hours per week. In comparison, the average 8–5 job has a 40-hour work week. A 40-hour work week translates into working 8 hours a day, Monday to Friday. Comparatively, a physician would work 12 hours a day for the same five days. This means less free time for the physician to pursue other interests or to spend with family and friends.

4. **Call**. Most residents are on-call 1 in 3 or 1 in 4. This means every third or fourth day (including through the night) they are responsible for patients. Call is usually taken from the hospital, meaning you sleep at the hospital the night you are on-call. In some rotations (surgery) it may be so busy that you do not sleep at all, but you are still expected to work the next day. Call *can* also be taken from home in some rotations (such as family medicine and psychiatry). These areas are usually not as busy.

In my opinion, call is the most demanding aspect of medicine—not only is it tiring, but it interferes with your lifestyle. If you are married it means that every third or fourth night you may not see your spouse. It also makes it difficult to plan activities in advance, or commit to an on-going activity on a specific day of the week.

Generally, call is less frequent after you have completed your residency; however, this varies considerably. The amount of call you are required to do depends on where you work and the number of other physicians in your group with whom you have made a deal to share call. For example, the only general practitioner in a small town would be

Other books in the *Life Line* series:

Opening the Doors to Canadian Medical Schools

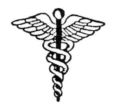

D. Roderick Elford, M.D.

Detselig Enterprises Ltd.
Calgary, Alberta

Opening the Doors to Canadian Medical Schools

© 1994 Rod Elford

Canadian Cataloguing in Publication Data

Elford, Rod, 19**

Opening the doors to Canadian medical schools

Includes bibliographical references.
ISBN 1-55059-084-7

1. Medical colleges–Canada–Entrance requirements. 2. Medical colleges–Canada–Entrance examinations. 3. Medical colleges–Canada–Directories. I. Title.
R749.A6E43 1994   610'.71'171   C94-910317-9

Publisher's Data

Detselig Enterprises Ltd. appreciates the financial support for our 1994 publishing program, provided by the Department of Communications, Canada Council and the Alberta Foundation for the Arts, a beneficiary of the Lottery Fund of the Government of Alberta.

Detselig Enterprises Ltd.
210, 1220 Kensington Road NW
Calgary, Alberta T2N 3P5

Edited by Sherry Wilson McEwen

Cover design by Dean MacDonald

Printed in Canada   ISBN 1-55059-084-7   SAN 115-0324

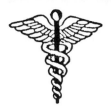

Chapter 7

Applying to Medical Schools

When and How to Apply

You have decided to apply for medical school—now what do you do? When do you apply? And how do you go about doing it?

APPLY EARLY

I recommend getting all the information (calendars and applications) from the medical schools to which you are thinking of applying, in the summer or early fall (a full year before you would be entering medical school). For example, collect all your information in the summer of 1995 if you are applying to start medical school in the fall of 1996. Get everything early, so you can leisurely browse through the material and make yourself aware of all important deadlines. (Most medical schools' deadlines for applications are late fall or early the following year.) To receive medical school calendars, write to the respective universities. Addresses for all of the Canadian medical schools can be found at the back of this book in Appendix A.

How Many Schools?

There are a number of factors to take into account when deciding how many schools to apply to. Generally, the "less competitive" you are compared to other applicants, the more schools you should apply to.

Play the odds! This means applying to schools at which you have the greatest chance of being accepted.

For example, if you are an average out-of-province candidate applying to schools with a strong preference for provincial or regional applicants, the competition for out-of-province applicants will be intense. Your best bet is to apply to schools which would look preferentially on your application, usually those closest to you. Table 15 in Appendix A gives information on the applicant preferences of each school.

Recommended Number of Applications

I recommend you apply to a minimum of three schools. (Be prepared to travel to any of the schools for an interview).

Table 9 on the opposite page lists the total number of first-year positions available in medical schools across the country, the number of people who applied, the number of applications per applicant, and the total number of applications received. During the last few years, there has been approximately four to five times as many applicants to medical school as there are positions. The total number of positions has been gradually decreasing since the early 1980s, mainly due to budget restraints, and will likely continue to drop slowly for the next few years. Conversely, the number of people applying to medical school is expected to continue to climb.

Time and Monetary Costs

Another factor that must be taken into account when applying to medical school is the cost. This includes not only the monetary cost of applying but the cost to your time. To apply to medical schools in Ontario, the base application fee is $150 plus $50 per school (there are five medical schools in Ontario). This means if you apply to one medical school in Ontario it will cost you $200, if you apply to two, it would be $250, etc. The application fee for other medical schools across the country varies but is approximately $50 per school. Just applying to a number of schools can add up. Secondly, the amount of time needed to fill in an application is substantial, although this varies widely, depending upon the application form for each school.

Table 9. Number of Canadian Medical School Positions and Applicants				
Year	Number of Positions	Number of Applicants	Applications per Applicant	Total Applicants
1992/93	1 732	8 259	2.55	21 091
1991/92	1 775	7 983	2.78	22 206
1990/91	1 791	7 768	2.75	21 374
1989/90	1 780	7 571	2.85	21 561
(*Canadian Medical Education Statistics 1993, Volume 15*. The Association of Canadian Medical Colleges, Ottawa, Canada, 1993, p.13,14,114,115,116)				

The application process is not standardized across the country. Some schools require one or more essays to be written with the first application. Other schools have a two-stage application process, whereby if you pass the first stage, you are required to send them more information. Whatever the procedure, completing forms is labor intensive and you should budget time accordingly. If possible, it is wise to take a lighter/easier course load your final year, so you will have extra time to fill out applications and/or go to interviews.

Conclusion

If practising medicine is a dream of yours, like all dreams in life, I believe you must pursue it to the best of your ability. Otherwise you will always wonder, what if . . . ?

Remember:

Do not give the admissions committee a reason to reject you.

Now, having read the main body of this book, go back to the original three answers you gave for wanting to become a doctor. Are they still the same? Or would you change anything?

If you have decided to pursue your goal of entering medical school, read through the Quick Reference as a review, then refer to the Appendices, which offer a basis for deciding to which schools you should apply.

One finger in the throat and one in the rectum makes a good diagnostician.
— Sir William Osler

Chapter 8

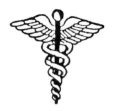

Quick Reference

This section is a brief review of all important points made in each chapter.

Summary of Academic Requirements

1. You must take the required courses. Generally this includes:
   - 1 year biology
   - 2 years chemistry
   - 1 year physics

   Check school calendar for specifics!
2. Strive for an average of at least 3.3 out of 4.0.
3. Take a major that you enjoy, not necessarily science.
4. Evenly distribute your workload (classes and labs).

Summary for MCAT

1. Get familiar with the exam style and questions— buy a manual or attend a course (I suggest the manual, it's cheaper).
2. Study adequately for the exam (start two months ahead).
3. Aim for an average score of 9 out of 15, or higher.
4. Try to get a good night's sleep before the test.

5. Write the MCAT in the spring, in most cases. It is best to write it at least 18 months before you plan to enter medical school.

6. Apply early to get your MCAT package—December to write the spring exam.

Summary for Essay

1. Answer the question.

2. Stay within the required length.

3. Make your essay memorable by incorporating personal examples. Have an exciting, attention-getting introduction, a logical, clear middle and a strong ending.

4. Make sure it looks neat and tidy on the page (it's typewritten). Have someone knowledgeable check it over for errors.

Summary for Interview

1. Be prepared mentally.

a) Know your interviewer.

b) Know the school.

c) Know how much they know about you.

d) Practise your interview personality.

e) Psyche yourself up for the interview.

2. Be prepared physically.

a) Be clean and well groomed.

b) Dress for success.

c) Try to be well rested.

3. Be prepared for antagonistic interviewers.

4. Arrange your interview schedule early.

Summary for Extra-curricular Activities

1. Get involved in extra-curricular activities you enjoy; activities that help you relax.
2. If possible, assume a leadership role.
3. Do not let your marks drop.

Summary for Reference Letter

1. Try to select referees that are well respected and/or politically important.
2. Make sure at least one of your professors gets to know you well.
3. Make sure the referees you select will write positive letters.

   Recommendation for three letters:

a) Two references from individuals who have an academic background (professors).
b) One additional reference from a person who has seen you perform at a high level of achievement, in a leadership position, or competently in a job/research situation.

When to Apply to Medical School

Get all your application packages early, preferably in the summer or early fall, at least a year before you would enter medical school. This means writing to the schools for information at least 18 months ahead of time.

To How Many Schools Should You Apply?

I recommend applying to at least three medical schools, to increase your chance of being accepted.

> *Medicine – the only profession that labours incessantly to destroy the reason for its own existence.*
> *– Anonymous*

Chapter 9

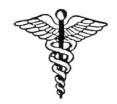

Other Considerations

What If You are Unsuccessful?

As the saying goes, "Do not put all your eggs in one basket." Although following the advice in this book will increase your odds of getting into medical school, it is not a guarantee. As was mentioned in an earlier section, it is wise to have a back-up plan in case you are not accepted.

If you are unsuccessful, what do you do? The answer to this question is either try again next year, or forget it. The final decision is up to you and indeed is a difficult one. There are a number of factors that must go into your decision, including how strongly you feel you want to be a doctor, why you were unsuccessful and determining if it is possible to change anything to make yourself more appealing to admissions committees. The official book put out by the Association of Canadian Medical Colleges states, "Other things being equal, chances for success of relatively uncompetitive candidates do not increase with the passage of time." (*Admission Requirements to Canadian Medical Colleges 1993/94*, p. 15) This does not mean you cannot make yourself more competitive. I know a doctor who applied eight times before he was accepted into medical school. This means it took him nine years before he finally realized his goal of getting into medical school!

Table 10 indicates the success rate of repeaters (people who applied before but did not get accepted) versus first-time applicants.

Table 10. Applicant Success Rates for Repeaters vs. Non-Repeaters (1992/93)			
Applicant Type	Number of Applicants	Number Admitted	Successful Applicants
Repeaters	2 792	613	22.0%
Non-repeaters	5 467	1 119	20.5%
Total	8 259	1 732	21.0%

(Canadian Medical Education Statistics 1993, Vol. 15. The Association of Canadian Medical Colleges, Ottawa, Canada, 1993, p.164)

The percentage of successful 1992/93 applicants who were repeaters was 613/1 732, or 35.4%. This means approximately one-third of all entrants to medical school in 1992-93 applied in earlier years and had been unsuccessful. Table 11 lists schools with the highest percentage of repeaters admitted.

Table 11. Schools that Admitted the Highest Percentage of Repeaters.			
1991-92		1992-93	
1. Alberta	53.4%	1. Queens	55.2%
2. Memorial	51.8%	2. Alberta	48.2%
3. UBC	47.9%	3. Memorial	47.3%

(Canadian Medical Education Statistics 1993, Volume 15. The Association of Canadian Medical Colleges, Ottawa, Canada, 1993, p.166).

What Do You Do For a Year?

If you are unsuccessful and do not get into medical school, what should you do for a year before you reapply? This is entirely up to you, however the majority of people I knew went back to school to: a) complete a degree, b) upgrade their marks in specific courses, c) boost their GPA by taking easy courses, or they d) rewrote the MCAT. Any one of these, or a combination, would likely improve your competitiveness. I have also known people who gained "life experience" either by working, (preferably in a health-related field), or taking a year off and travelling.

> *The hardest thing to learn in life is which bridge to cross and which to burn.*
> *– David Russel*

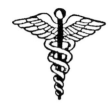

Chapter 10

Foreign Applicants

Although this book was written as a guide for Canadian citizens or landed immigrants, I did do some research regarding the success of foreign applicants. Since a number of Canadian medical schools' tuition fees are relatively inexpensive compared to medical schools in other countries (see Table 16 in Appendix A), a substantial number of foreign citizens apply annually to Canadian schools. Table 12 on the following page shows that the number of foreign, as well as the total applicants, has increased over the last few years. In 1992/93 foreign applicants made up 514 out of 8 259 total applicants (6.2%).

Success Rates for Foreign Applicants

Table 13 on the following page indicates the percentage success rate for applicants who fall within each citizen class. For example, of the 514 foreign applicants in 1992/93, 7.2% (37 people) were accepted to a Canadian medical school. Canadian citizens on the other hand, had a success rate of 22.3%, or approximately three times greater than a foreign applicant.

Although the success rate for foreign students is low, some applicants do get accepted. Unfortunately, as education funding is cut further by the federal and provincial governments, the forecast becomes increasingly gloomier for foreigners wanting entrance to any post-secondary programs in Canada. Additionally, tuition fees may rise substantially.

Table 12. Applicant Numbers Based on Citizenship

Year	Canadian Citizens	Landed Immigrants	Foreign Citizens	Total Applicants
1992/93	7 230	515	514	8 259
1991/92	7 063	468	452	7 983
1990/91	6 875	424	469	7 768
1989/90	6 768	392	411	7 571

(*Canadian Medical Education Statistics 1993, Vol. 15*. The Association of Canadian Medical Colleges, Ottawa, Canada, 1993, p.130)

Table 13. Relative Opportunities (Success Rates) for the Study of Medicine

Year	Canadian Citizens	Landed Immigrants	Foreign Citizens
1992/93	22.3%	15.7%	7.2%
1991/92	23.1%	19.9%	7.7%
1990/91	23.9%	20.3%	7.2%
1989/90	24.6%	20.4%	5.1%

(*Canadian Medical Education Statistics 1993, Vol. 15*. The Association of Medical Colleges, Ottawa, Canada, 1993, p. 124, 125)

Medical School Specifics

"Medical School Specifics" contains a large amount of information and statistics in table form. This section gives you information about each medical school and its applicants. Take some time to go through the tables.

Note: All dollar figures are in Canadian currency.

The majority of the data in the tables is from a manual entitled, *Admission Requirements for Canadian Medical Schools*. If you are interested in this book, it can be purchased from the Association of Canadian Medical Colleges (address can be found in the section "Other Helpful Addresses" in this appendix). Alternatively, the Journal of the American Medical Association included similar information in a summary of all American and Canadian medical schools in their September 1, 1993 issue. (JAMA, Volume 270, No. 9)

> *A physician is a person who works sixteen hours a day telling people to slow down or they'll get high blood pressure.*
> *– Anonymous*

Table 14. Canadian Medical School Characteristics

University	Location (city)	Founded	Program Length	Program Language	Owner-ship
British Columbia	Vancouver, B.C.	1950	4 years	English	public
Calgary	Calgary, Alta.	1970	3 years	English	public
Alberta	Edmonton, Alta.	1913	4 years	English	public
Saskat-chewan	Saskatoon, Sask.	1953	4 years	English	public
Manitoba	Winnipeg, MB	1883	4 years	English	public
Western	London, Ont.	1882	4 years	English	private
McMaster	Hamilton, Ont.	1969	3 years	English	private
Toronto	Toronto, Ont.	1843	4 years	English	public
Queens	Kingston, Ont.	1854	4 years	English	private
Ottawa	Ottawa, Ont.	1945	4 years	English	private
McGill	Montreal, Que.	1829	4 years	English	private
Montreal	Montreal, Que.	1877	4 years	French	private
Sherbrooke	Sherbrooke, Que.	1966	4 years	French	private
Laval	Quebec, Que.	1852	4 years	French	private
Dalhousie	Halifax, N.S.	1868	4 years	English	private
Memorial	St. John's, Nfld.	1925	4 years	English	public

Table 15. Medical School Class Size, Total Applicants, Preferences

University	Class Size (1993)	Total 1992/93 Applicants	Applicant Preference
British Columbia	120	558	BC residents
Calgary	69	671	Alberta residents
Alberta	110 + 2*	765	Alta. residents
Saskatchewan	60	391	Saskatchewan residents
Manitoba	70	300	Manitoba residents
Western	96	2 046	no preference
McMaster	100	2 628	preference for surrounding area
Toronto	177	1 998	Ontario residents
Queens	75	1 246	no preference
Ottawa	84	1 990	preference for surrounding area
McGill	140	1 352**	no preference
Montreal	180	2 046	Quebec residents
Sherbrooke	105	1 944	Quebec residents
Laval	146	1 919	Quebec residents
Dalhousie	82	673	Maritimes resident
Memorial	56	564	Newfoundland & New Brunswick residents

*Two positions are reserved for native students; in the event they are not filled, the positions remain vacant.
**McGill admits some students to a pre-medicine program. If their progress is satisfactory, these candidates continue on in the four-year program.

Table 16. University Tuition, Student Intern Stipends and Resident Salaries

University	Tuition (1993) for Canadians	Foreign Students Tuition	Other Fees	Student Stipend	PGY-1 Salary
British Columbia	$3 501	—	$153	$5 652	$34 268
Calgary	$3 604	$7 208	$289	$3 600	$30 556
Alberta	$3 165	$6 331	ncluded	$3 600	$30 556
Saskat-chewan	$3 990	—	$75	$5 400	$30 351
Manitoba	$3 775	$3 775	$77	$3 886	$30 417
Western	$2 576	$12 454	$664	$1 724	$36 075
McMaster	$3 865	$17 750	$328	$1 724	$36 075
Toronto	$2 576	$12 454	$389	$1 724	$36 075
Queens	$2 576	$11 891	$432	$1 724	$36 075
Ottawa	$2 576	—	$236	$1 724	$36 075
McGill	$2 145	$7 901	included	$0	$33 264
Montreal	$2 124	$7 584	$30	$0	$33 264
Sherbrooke	$2 574	$11 256	$380	$0	$33 264
Laval	$2 550	$11 232	$277	$0	$33 264
Dalhousie	$3 465	$5 165	$212	$2 592	$31 457
Memorial	$1 700 (Yr. 1,2) $2 550 (Yr. 3,4)	$1 275 $3 825	$50 $75	$3 465	$30 176

Student stipend = the amount paid a medical student during his/her clerkship year.
PGY-1 Salary = (post-graduate year one) the amount paid to a physician the first year out of medical school. Salaries are negotiated by each provincial medical association. Some provinces are in the process of negotiating new contracts. These values are accurate as of January 1994.

University	Amount in 1991	Rank in 1991	Rank in 1990	Rank in 1989	Rank in 1988
Table 17. Research Spending at Canadian Medical Schools					
Toronto	1 49 585 000	1	1	1	1
McGill	1 04 084 000	2	2	2	2
Montreal	91 134 000	3	3	3	3
Laval	59 114 000	4	8	10	9
Alberta	43 426 000	5	4	4	4
British Columbia	41 989 000	6	5	7	6
McMaster	41 632 000	7	6	6	5
Western	38 644 000	8	7	5	7
Calgary	36 859 000	9	9	8	8
Ottawa	33 983 000	10	11	9	11
Manitoba	27 552 000	11	10	11	10
Sherbrooke	21 517 000	12	13	13	13
Queens	21 449 000	13	12	12	12
Dalhousie	13 486 000	14	14	14	14
Saskatchewan	13 021 000	15	15	15	15
Memorial	4 994 000	16	16	16	16

Statistics on Medical School Applicants

There are a number of interesting trends occurring in medical schools.

1. Decreasing number of positions available for medical school

The total number of entrants to medical school increased steadily from 1 011 students in 1957/58 to a peak of 1 887 in 1980/81 and 1983/84. But the number of entrants has slowly declined during the last decade, falling to 1 732 in 1992/93. This number is expected to decline even further over the next few years due to budget cuts.

2. Increasing number of women as a percentage of medical school class

The number of women being accepted to medical school has also increased significantly from 10.3% of the entering class in 1960/61, 20.2% in 1970/71, 40.0% in 1980/81, and in 1993/94 surpassed men with 51%.

TABLE 18. Top Three Schools with the Highest Percentage of Female Students		
Medical School	**% of Women Medical Students, All Years**	**% of Women Medical Students in Entering Class, 1992/93**
McMaster	64.7	61.0
Memorial	47.3	46.4
Dalhousie	43.4	52.3

3. Increasing older age of students entering medical school

Older students (>26 years) are becoming a larger proportion of those entering medical classes. Older students made up 5.8% of all entrants in 1977/78 rising to 20.4% in 1992/93.

Table 19. Age of Successful Applicants				
Percentage of Entrants in Age Group				
Year	**<20**	**20-22**	**23-26**	**>26**
1993	14.5	36.3	28.8	20.4
1992	17.0	47.4	23.5	12.1
1991	18.3	46.4	24.5	10.8
1978	23.8	49.4	21.0	5.8

Canadian Medical School Addresses

University of British Columbia
Faculty of Medicine
2194 Health Sciences Center Mall
Vancouver, British Columbia
V6T 1W5
(604) 228-2421

University of Calgary
Faculty of Medicine
3330 Hospital Drive N.W.
Calgary, Alberta
T2N 4N1
(403) 220-6541

University of Alberta
Faculty of Medicine
W.C. Mackenzie Building
Edmonton, Alberta
T6G 2R7
(403) 492-6621

University of Saskatchewan
Faculty of Medicine
B103, Health Sciences Building
Saskatoon, Saskatchewan
S7N 0W0
(306) 966-6135

University of Manitoba
Faculty of Medicine
753 McDermot Avenue
Winnipeg, Manitoba
R3E 0W3
(204) 788-6557

University of Western Ontario
Faculty of Medicine
London, Ontario
N6A 5C1
(514) 661-2075

McMaster University
Faculty of Medicine
1200 Main Street West
Hamilton, Ontario
L8N 3Z5
(416) 525-9140

University of Toronto
Faculty of Medicine
King's College Circle
Toronto, Ontario
M5S 1A8
(416) 978-2710

Queens' University
Faculty of Medicine
Kingston, Ontario
K7L 3N6
(613) 545-2544

University of Ottawa
School of Medicine
Ottawa, Ontario
K1H 8M5
(613) 787-6400

McGill University
Faculty of Medicine
3655 Drummond Street
Montreal, Québec
H3G 1Y6
(514) 398-3515

Université de Montreal
Faculté de Médecine
P.O. Box 6207, Station A
Montreal, Quebec
H3C 3J7
(514) 343-6305

Université de Sherbrooke
Faculté de Médecine
Sherbrooke, Québec
J1H 5N4
(819) 564-5200

Université Laval
Faculté de Médecine
Québec, Québec
G1K 7P4
(418) 656-2131

Dalhousie Universiy
Faculty of Medicine
Sir Charles Tupper Medical Building
Halifax, Nova Scotia
B3H 4H7
(902) 492-3591

Memorial University
Faculty of Medicine
Health Sciences Center
Prince Phillip Drive
St. John's, Newfoundland
A1B 3V6
(709) 737-6602

Other Helpful Addresses

Admission Requirements for Canadian Medical
Schools
Association of Canadian Medical Colleges
151 Slater Street, Suite 1006
Ottawa, Ontario K1P 5N1

American Association of Medical Colleges
2450 North Street N.W.
Washington, D.C. 20037-1126
(202) 828-0416

Canadian Medical Association
P.O. Box 8650
Ottawa, Ontario K1G 0G8
(613) 731-9331

Canadian Medical Education Statistics
Association of Canadian Medical Colleges
151 Slater Street, Suite 1006
Ottawa, Ontario K1P 5N1

College of Family Physicians of Canada
4000 Leslie Street
Willowdale, Ontario M2K 2R9
(416) 493-7513

MCAT Membership and Subscriptions
Association of American Medical Colleges
One Dupont Circle, N.W.
Washington, D.C. 20036

Royal College of Physicians and Surgeons
of Canada
74 Stanley Avenue
Ottawa, Ontario K1M 1P4
(613) 746-8177

Ethics of Medicine

This appendix contains the following statements of ethical conduct for physicians, surgeons and medical students:

- The Hippocratic Oath
- Code of Ethics for Undergraduate Medical Students
- Canadian Medical Association Code of Ethics

> *The life so short, the art so long to learn, opportunity fleeting, experience treacherous, judgement difficult.*
> *– Hippocrates (on medicine)*

> *The unexamined life is not worth living.*
> *– Socrates*

The Hippocratic Oath

I swear by Apollo the physician, by Aesculapius, Hygeia, and Panacea, and I take to witness all the gods, all the goddesses, to keep according to my ability and my judgement the following Oath:

To consider dear to me as my parents him who taught me this art; to live in common with him and if necessary to share my goods with him; to look upon his children as my own brothers, to teach them this art if they so desire without fee or written promise; to impart to my sons and the sons of the master who taught me and the disciples who have enrolled themselves and have agreed to the rules of the profession, but to these alone, the precepts and the instruction. I will prescribe regimen for the good of my patients according to my ability and my judgement and never do harm to anyone. To please no one will I prescribe a deadly drug. Nor give advice which will cause his death. Nor will I give a woman a pessary to procure abortion. But I will preserve the purity of my life and my art. I will not cut for stone, even for patients in whom this disease is manifest; I will leave this operation to be performed by practitioners (specialists in this art). In every house where I come I will enter only for the good of my patients, keeping myself from the pleasure of love with women or with men, be they free or slaves. All that may come to my knowledge in the exercise of my profession or outside of my profession or in daily commerce with men, which ought not to be spread abroad, I will keep secret and never reveal. If I keep this oath faithfully, may I enjoy my life and practice my art, respected by all men and in all times; but if I swerve from it or violate it, may the reverse be my lot.

Code of Ethics
for Undergraduate Medical Students

Declaration of Geneva

(Adopted by the General Assembly of the World Medical Association at Geneva, Switzerland, September, 1948)

At the time of being admitted as member of the medical profession:

I solemnly pledge, myself to consecrate my life to the service of humanity,

I will give to my teachers the respect and gratitude which is their due;

I will practice my profession with conscience and dignity; the health of my patient will be my first consideration.

I will respect the secrets which are confided in me; I will maintain by all the means in my power, the honor and the noble tradition of the medical profession;

My colleagues will be my brothers; I will not permit consideration of religion, nationality, race, party politics, or social standing to intervene between my duty and my patient;

I will maintain the utmost respect for human life from the time of conception; even under threat, I will not use my medical knowledge contrary to the laws of humanity.

I make these promises solemnly, freely and upon my honor.

The Canadian Medical Association Code of Ethics

Principles of Ethical Behavior for all physicians, including those who may not be engaged directly in clinical practice.

I

Consider first the well-being of the patient.

II

Honour your profession
and its traditions.

III

Recognize your limitations
and the special skills of others in the prevention and
treatment of disease.

IV

Protect the patient's secrets.

V

Teach and be taught.

VI

Remember that integrity
and professional ability should be
your only advertisement.

VII

Be responsible in
setting a value on your services.

References

American Association of Medical Colleges. *Directory of American Medical Education 1991-1992, 38th Edition*. Washington, D.C. 1991.

Association of American Medical Colleges. *Medical School Admission Requirements (U.S. and Canada) 1994-95*. Washington D.C. 1993.

Association of American Medical Colleges. *Medical College Admissions Test 1993 Registration Packet*. Washington, D.C. 1993.

American Medical Association. *Physician Market Place Statistics 1991*. Chicago: 1991.

Canadian Medical School Calendars 1992/93. University of British Columbia, University of Alberta, University of Calgary, University of Saskatchewan, University of Manitoba, University of Western Ontario, McMaster University, University of Toronto, Queens University, University of Ottawa, McGill University, Université Laval, Université de Montreal, Université de Sherbrooke, University of Dalhousie, Memorial University.

Department of National Health and Welfare, Health Information Division. *Earnings of Physicians and Dentists in Canada*. Ottawa: 1990.

Medical Schools in Canada – Appendix 1B. *Journal of the American Medical Association*. 270, 9 (Sept. 1 1993): 1113–1115.

Royal College of Physicians and Surgeons of Canada. *Accredited Residency Programs*. Ottawa: 1992.

The Association of Canadian Medical Colleges. *Admission Requirements to Canadian Faculties of Medicine and their Selection Policies 1993/94 & 1994/95.* Ottawa: 1992.

The Association of Canadian Medical Colleges. *Canadian Medical Education Statistics 1993. Vol. 15.* Ottawa: 1993.

COMMITTED TO THE DEVELOPMENT OF CULTURE AND THE ARTS